GOUT DIET COOKBOOK FOR SENIORS

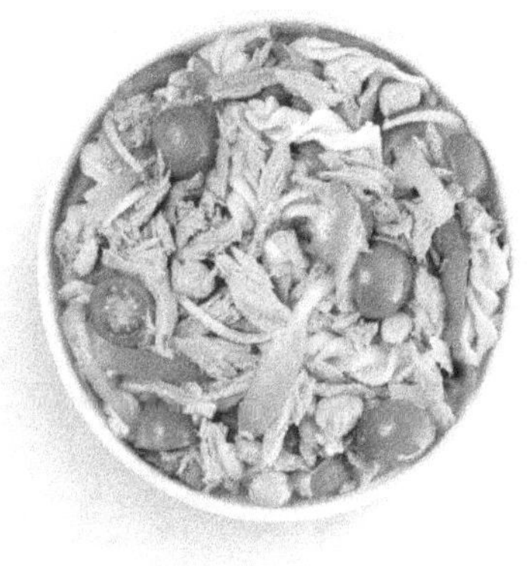

DR. JESSICA SMITH

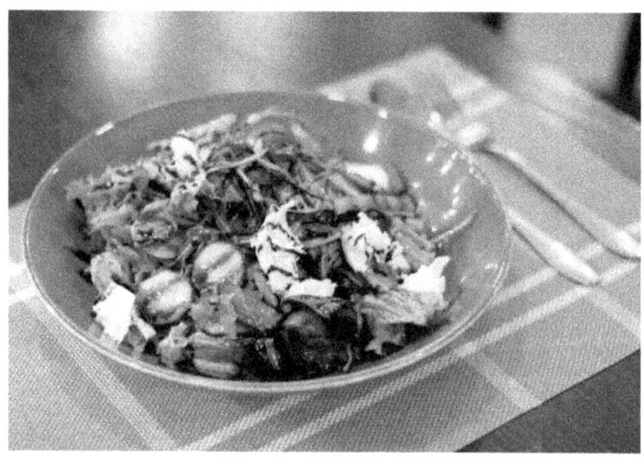

CHAPTER ONE

How to Use this Cookbook

Educate Yourself: Start by understanding what gout is and how it affects your body. Learn about foods that are high in purines, as they can exacerbate gout symptoms. Common high-purine foods include red meat, organ meats, and certain seafood.

Consult a Dietitian: Before making any significant changes to your diet, consult a registered dietitian or healthcare professional. They can provide personalized advice based on your specific health needs and dietary restrictions.

Focus on Hydration: Staying hydrated is crucial for managing gout. Aim to drink at least 8 glasses of water per day to help flush out uric acid from your body.

Emphasize Low-Purine Foods: Base your meals around foods that are low in purines, such as fruits, vegetables, whole grains, and low-fat dairy products. Incorporate plenty of leafy greens, berries, nuts, and legumes into your diet.

Limit High-Purine Foods: While it's not necessary to completely eliminate high-purine foods, it's important to consume them in moderation. Limit your intake of red meat, game meats, shellfish, and certain types of fish like anchovies and sardines.

Choose Lean Protein Sources: Opt for lean sources of protein such as poultry, tofu, eggs, and legumes. These options are lower in purines compared to red meat and can still provide essential nutrients.

Watch Your Alcohol Intake: Alcohol, especially beer and spirits, can increase uric acid levels in the body and trigger gout attacks. Limit your alcohol consumption, and if you do drink, opt for moderate amounts of wine or beer.

Experiment with Flavorful Herbs and Spices: Use herbs and spices to add flavor to your meals without relying on high-purine ingredients like salt and rich sauces. Experiment with fresh herbs like basil, cilantro, and parsley, as well as spices such as turmeric, cumin, and ginger.

Plan Balanced Meals: Aim for balanced meals that include a variety of nutrients. Incorporate a mix of carbohydrates, protein, and healthy fats into each meal to help maintain stable blood sugar levels and promote overall health.

Keep Portions in Check: Pay attention to portion sizes to prevent overeating, which can contribute to weight gain and increase the risk of gout attacks. Use smaller plates, measure out servings, and practice mindful eating to avoid consuming more than your body needs.

Understanding Gout Diet for Seniors

Understanding the gout diet for seniors is crucial for managing this painful condition effectively. Gout is a form of arthritis caused by the accumulation of uric acid crystals in the joints, leading to inflammation, swelling, and intense pain, especially in the joints of the feet, ankles, and knees.

Seniors are particularly susceptible to gout due to factors such as decreased kidney function, medication use, and lifestyle choices.

The gout diet for seniors focuses on reducing the intake of foods high in purines, as purines break down into uric acid in the body.

These foods include red meat, organ meats, shellfish, and certain types of fish like anchovies and sardines. Instead, seniors are encouraged to consume low-purine foods such as fruits, vegetables, whole grains, lean proteins like poultry and tofu, and low-fat dairy products.

Hydration is also a key aspect of the gout diet for seniors, as it helps to flush out excess uric acid from the body. Seniors should aim to drink plenty of water throughout the day and limit alcohol consumption, as alcohol can increase uric acid levels.

Additionally, seniors with gout should maintain a healthy weight through regular exercise and portion control to reduce the risk of gout flare-ups.

Overall, understanding and adhering to the gout diet can significantly improve the quality of life for seniors living with this condition.

Principles of Gout Diet for Seniors

The principles of the gout diet for seniors revolve around managing uric acid levels in the body to prevent gout flare-ups and minimize the associated pain and discomfort.

Here are some key principles:

Limit High-Purine Foods: Seniors with gout should reduce their intake of foods high in purines, as these substances break down into uric acid. High-purine foods include red meat, organ meats (such as liver and kidneys), shellfish, and certain types of fish (like anchovies and sardines).

Focus on Low-Purine Foods: Emphasize the consumption of low-purine foods, such as fruits, vegetables, whole grains, legumes, nuts, seeds, low-fat dairy products, and lean proteins like poultry, tofu, and eggs. These foods help maintain a balanced diet while minimizing uric acid production.

Stay Hydrated: Adequate hydration is crucial for seniors with gout, as it helps to flush out excess uric acid from the body through urine. Encourage seniors to drink plenty of water throughout the day, aiming for at least eight glasses or more depending on individual needs.

Moderate Alcohol Intake: Alcohol consumption can contribute to elevated uric acid levels, so seniors with gout should limit their intake of alcoholic beverages, particularly beer and spirits.

Maintain a Healthy Weight: Excess weight can exacerbate gout symptoms, so seniors should aim to maintain a healthy weight through a balanced diet and regular exercise.

The gout diet offers numerous benefits for seniors, helping them manage their condition effectively and improve their overall quality of life.

Here are some of the key benefits:

Reduced Pain and Inflammation: Following a gout diet can help seniors reduce the frequency and severity of gout flare-ups, leading to decreased pain and inflammation in the joints.

By avoiding foods high in purines, seniors can lower their uric acid levels and minimize the risk of crystal formation in the joints.

Improved Joint Health: By adhering to the gout diet, seniors can maintain better joint health and mobility. The diet encourages the consumption of anti-inflammatory foods, such as fruits, vegetables, and whole grains, which can help alleviate joint stiffness and discomfort associated with gout.

Better Management of Chronic Conditions: Seniors with gout often have other chronic conditions, such as hypertension, diabetes, and cardiovascular disease. The gout diet emphasizes healthy eating habits, including the consumption of low-fat dairy, lean proteins, and whole grains, which can help seniors better manage these comorbidities.

Enhanced Kidney Function: Since gout is associated with elevated uric acid levels, following a gout diet can reduce the strain on the kidneys by preventing the formation of uric acid crystals. This can lead to improved kidney function and decreased risk of kidney stones or other renal complications.

Overall Health and Well-being: By adopting a gout diet, seniors can enjoy better overall health and well-being. A balanced diet rich in fruits, vegetables, and lean proteins can provide essential nutrients, vitamins, and minerals necessary for optimal health, while also supporting healthy aging and longevity.

In conclusion, the gout diet offers a multitude of benefits for seniors, ranging from reduced pain and inflammation to improved joint health, better management of chronic conditions, enhanced kidney function, and overall improved health and well-being.

By making simple dietary modifications, seniors can effectively manage their gout and enjoy a higher quality of life.

Tips for Gout Diet for Seniors

Managing gout through dietary modifications can be simplified with these practical tips tailored for seniors:

Educate and Plan: Seniors should learn about foods high in purines and plan their meals accordingly. Keeping a food diary can help identify triggers and track dietary patterns.

Hydration: Encourage seniors to drink plenty of water throughout the day to help flush out uric acid from the body. Herbal teas and infused water can add variety while maintaining hydration.

Portion Control: While low-purine foods are encouraged, portion control is key. Seniors should be mindful of serving sizes to prevent overconsumption of purine-rich foods like red meat or seafood.

Include Anti-Inflammatory Foods: Emphasize incorporating anti-inflammatory foods such as berries, cherries, leafy greens, and fatty fish like salmon into their diet to help reduce inflammation and manage gout symptoms.

Limit Alcohol and Sugary Beverages: Alcohol, especially beer and spirits, can exacerbate gout symptoms. Seniors should limit alcohol consumption and opt for water, herbal teas, or low-sugar beverages instead.

Choose Low-Fat Dairy: Low-fat dairy products like milk, yogurt, and cheese can be included in moderation as they may help lower uric acid levels.

Healthy Fats: Encourage the consumption of healthy fats found in avocados, nuts, seeds, and olive oil, which can help reduce inflammation and support overall health.

Consult a Healthcare Professional: Seniors should consult with a healthcare provider or dietitian to tailor the gout diet to their individual needs and ensure it aligns with any other medical conditions or medications they may have.

By implementing these tips, seniors can effectively manage their gout through dietary modifications while enjoying flavorful and nourishing meals.

Guidelines for Gout Diet for Seniors

For seniors managing gout, adhering to specific guidelines can help control symptoms and improve overall health.

Here are essential guidelines for a gout diet tailored to seniors:

Limit High-Purine Foods: Seniors should reduce intake of foods high in purines, such as red meat, organ meats, shellfish, and certain types of fish like anchovies and sardines. These foods contribute to increased uric acid levels in the body.

Focus on Low-Purine Options: Emphasize consuming low-purine foods, including fruits, vegetables, whole grains, legumes, nuts, seeds, low-fat dairy products, and lean proteins like poultry and tofu.

These options provide essential nutrients without raising uric acid levels significantly.

Stay Hydrated: Seniors should maintain proper hydration by drinking plenty of water throughout the day. Adequate hydration helps flush out uric acid from the body, reducing the risk of gout flare-ups.

Moderate Alcohol Consumption: Limiting alcohol intake, especially beer and spirits, can help manage gout symptoms. Alcohol consumption can increase uric acid levels, leading to gout attacks.

Manage Weight: Seniors should aim to maintain a healthy weight through a balanced diet and regular exercise. Excess weight can contribute to gout flare-ups and joint pain.

Monitor Portion Sizes: Seniors should be mindful of portion sizes, especially when consuming high-purine foods. Controlling portion sizes can help prevent overconsumption of purines.

Consult Healthcare Provider: Seniors should consult with a healthcare provider or dietitian to develop a personalized gout diet plan tailored to their individual needs and medical history.

By following these guidelines, seniors can effectively manage gout and reduce the frequency and severity of gout attacks, leading to improved overall health and well-being.

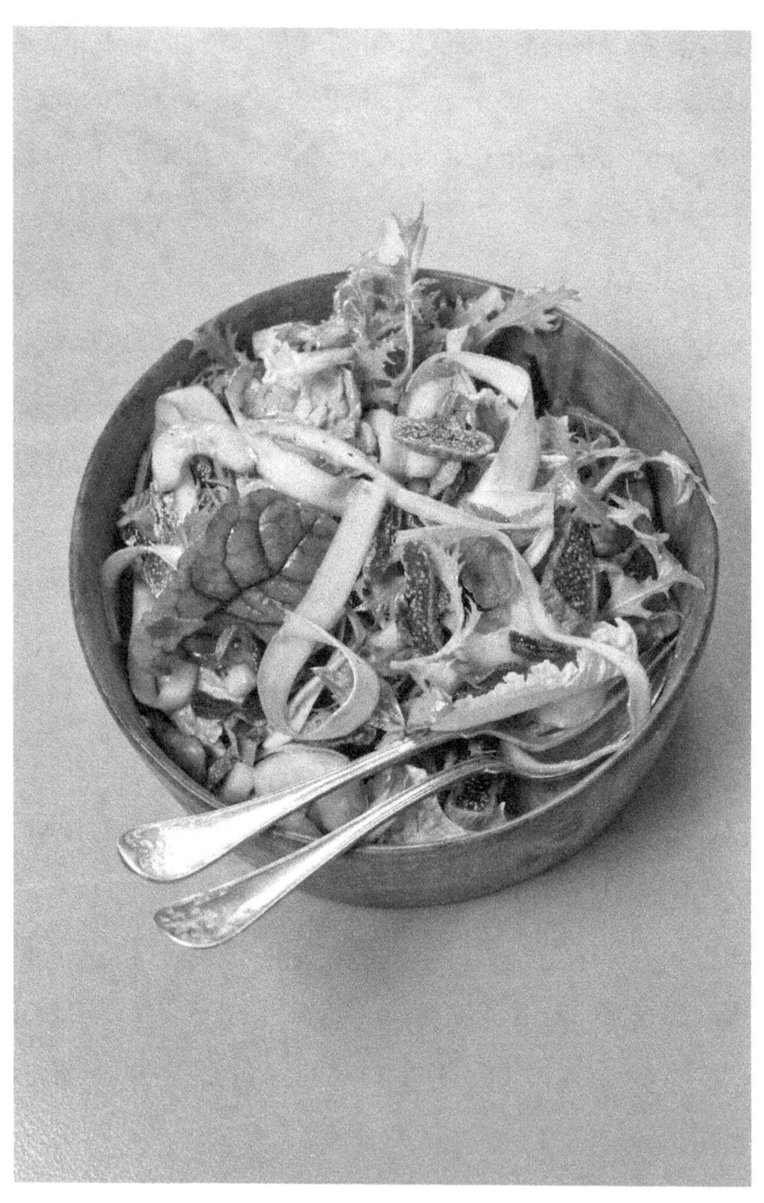

CHAPTER TWO

1. Berry Oatmeal

Ingredients:

* 1/2 cup rolled oats

* 1 cup water or milk (dairy or plant-based)

* 1/2 cup mixed berries (such as strawberries, blueberries, raspberries)

* 1 tablespoon honey or maple syrup (optional)

* 1 tablespoon chopped nuts or seeds (optional)

Instructions:

* In a saucepan, bring water or milk to a boil.

* Stir in rolled oats and reduce heat to simmer. Cook for 5-7 minutes, stirring occasionally, until oats are creamy.

* Remove from heat and stir in mixed berries.

* Sweeten with honey or maple syrup if desired.

* Sprinkle with chopped nuts or seeds for added crunch.

* Serve hot and enjoy!

Health Benefits:

* This breakfast is rich in fiber from oats and antioxidants from mixed berries, promoting heart health, digestion, and inflammation reduction.

Preparation Time: 10 minutes

2. Avocado Toast with Poached Egg

Ingredients:

* 1 ripe avocado
* 2 slices whole-grain bread, toasted
* 2 eggs
* Salt and pepper to taste
* Optional toppings: sliced tomatoes, feta cheese, or red pepper flakes

Instructions:

* Mash avocado in a bowl and season with salt and pepper.
* Poach eggs in simmering water for 3-4 minutes until whites are set but yolks are still runny.

* Spread mashed avocado evenly on toasted bread slices.

* Top each slice with a poached egg.

* Add optional toppings as desired.

* Serve immediately.

Health Benefits:

* Avocado provides healthy fats, while whole-grain bread offers fiber.

* Eggs are a good source of protein, supporting muscle health.

Preparation Time: 15 minutes

3. Greek Yogurt Parfait

Ingredients:

* 1 cup Greek yogurt (plain or flavored)

* 1/2 cup mixed berries (such as strawberries, blueberries, raspberries)

* 1/4 cup granola

* 1 tablespoon honey or maple syrup (optional)

Instructions:

* In a serving glass or bowl, layer Greek yogurt, mixed berries, and granola.
* Repeat the layers until ingredients are used up.
* Drizzle with honey or maple syrup if desired.
* Serve immediately as a nutritious and filling breakfast option.

Health Benefits:

* Greek yogurt provides probiotics for gut health, while berries offer antioxidants and fiber.
* Granola adds crunch and energy.

Preparation Time: 5 minutes

4. Spinach and Mushroom Omelette

Ingredients:

* 2 eggs
* 1/4 cup baby spinach leaves
* 1/4 cup sliced mushrooms
* 1 tablespoon olive oil
* Salt and pepper to taste

* Optional: shredded cheese or diced tomatoes

Instructions:

* In a bowl, beat eggs and season with salt and pepper.
* Heat olive oil in a non-stick skillet over medium heat.
* Add mushrooms and sauté until tender, then add spinach and cook until wilted.
* Pour beaten eggs into the skillet, swirling to evenly distribute.
* Cook until edges start to set, then gently lift edges with a spatula to let uncooked egg flow underneath.
* Once the omelette is almost set, sprinkle with optional cheese or tomatoes.
* Fold omelette in half and cook for another minute until cheese melts.
* Slide onto a plate and serve hot.

Health Benefits:

* This omelette is packed with protein from eggs and nutrients from spinach and mushrooms, supporting overall health and immunity.

Preparation Time: 10 minutes

Ingredients:

* 1 ripe banana
* 1/2 cup Greek yogurt (plain or flavored)
* 1/4 cup walnuts
* 1/2 cup milk (dairy or plant-based)
* 1 tablespoon honey or maple syrup (optional)
* Ice cubes (optional)

Instructions:

* In a blender, combine banana, Greek yogurt, walnuts, milk, and honey or maple syrup.
* Blend until smooth and creamy.
* Add ice cubes if desired for a colder consistency.
* Pour into a glass and garnish with a sprinkle of chopped walnuts.
* Serve immediately as a refreshing and nutritious breakfast option.

Health Benefits:

* This smoothie is rich in potassium from banana and omega-3 fatty acids from walnuts, supporting heart health and inflammation reduction.

Preparation Time: 5 minutes

6. Quinoa Breakfast Bowl

Ingredients:

* 1/2 cup cooked quinoa
* 1/4 cup sliced strawberries
* 1/4 cup blueberries
* 1 tablespoon honey or maple syrup
* 1 tablespoon chopped almonds or pecans
* 1/4 teaspoon cinnamon (optional)

Instructions:

* In a bowl, combine cooked quinoa, sliced strawberries, and blueberries.
* Drizzle with honey or maple syrup and sprinkle with chopped nuts.
* Add a pinch of cinnamon if desired for extra flavor.

* Stir gently to combine all ingredients.
* Serve warm or cold as a nutrient-packed breakfast bowl.

Health Benefits:

* Quinoa offers protein and fiber, while berries provide antioxidants and vitamins.
* Nuts add healthy fats and crunch.

Preparation Time: 10 minutes

7. Veggie Breakfast Burrito

Ingredients:

* 2 eggs, beaten
* 1/4 cup diced bell peppers
* 1/4 cup diced onions
* 1/4 cup diced tomatoes
* 2 tablespoons chopped cilantro
* 2 whole wheat tortillas
* Salt and pepper to taste
* Cooking spray

Instructions:

* In a skillet, heat cooking spray over medium heat.
* Add diced bell peppers and onions, sauté until softened.
* Pour beaten eggs into the skillet and scramble until cooked through.
* Stir in diced tomatoes and chopped cilantro, season with salt and pepper.
* Warm tortillas in the microwave or on a skillet.
* Spoon egg mixture onto each tortilla and roll up to form burritos.
* Serve immediately, optionally with salsa or avocado slices on the side.

Health Benefits:

* This veggie-packed burrito provides fiber, vitamins, and minerals essential for seniors' health, promoting digestion and immune function.

Preparation Time: 15 minutes

8. Cottage Cheese and Fruit Bowl

Ingredients:

* 1/2 cup low-fat cottage cheese
* 1/2 cup sliced peaches or pineapple chunks (fresh or canned in juice)
* 1/4 cup sliced almonds or sunflower seeds
* 1 tablespoon honey or maple syrup (optional)

Instructions:

* In a bowl, spoon cottage cheese.
* Top with sliced peaches or pineapple chunks.
* Sprinkle with sliced almonds or sunflower seeds.
* Drizzle with honey or maple syrup if desired for added sweetness.
* Serve immediately as a refreshing and protein-rich breakfast option.

Health Benefits:

* Cottage cheese offers protein and calcium, while fruits provide vitamins and antioxidants.
* Nuts or seeds add healthy fats and crunch.

Preparation Time: 5 minutes

9. Overnight Chia Pudding

Ingredients:

* 2 tablespoons chia seeds

* 1/2 cup almond milk or any milk of choice

* 1/4 teaspoon vanilla extract

* 1 tablespoon honey or maple syrup

* Sliced strawberries or blueberries for topping

Instructions:

* In a bowl or jar, combine chia seeds, almond milk, vanilla extract, and honey or maple syrup.

* Stir well to combine all ingredients.

* Cover and refrigerate overnight or for at least 4 hours until mixture thickens.

* Stir again before serving and top with sliced strawberries or blueberries.

* Enjoy chilled as a nutritious and filling breakfast option.

Health Benefits:

* Chia seeds are rich in fiber and omega-3 fatty acids, promoting heart health and digestion.
* Almond milk provides calcium and vitamin D.

Preparation Time: 5 minutes (plus overnight chilling)

10. Vegetable Frittata

Ingredients:

* 4 eggs
* 1/2 cup diced bell peppers
* 1/2 cup diced onions
* 1/2 cup chopped spinach
* 1/4 cup shredded mozzarella cheese
* Salt and pepper to taste
* Cooking spray

Instructions:

* Preheat the oven to 350°F (175°C).
* In a bowl, whisk together eggs, salt, and pepper.
* Heat cooking spray in an oven-safe skillet over medium heat.

* Add diced bell peppers and onions, sauté until softened.

* Stir in chopped spinach and cook until wilted.

* Pour whisked eggs over the vegetables in the skillet.

* Sprinkle shredded mozzarella cheese on top.

* Transfer the skillet to the preheated oven and bake for 12-15 minutes, or until eggs are set and cheese is melted.

* Remove from the oven and let it cool slightly before slicing.

* Serve warm as a protein-packed breakfast option.

Health Benefits:

* This vegetable frittata provides protein and vitamins from eggs and vegetables, supporting muscle health and immunity.

Preparation Time: 20 minutes

1. Grilled Chicken Salad

Ingredients:

* 1 grilled chicken breast, sliced
* 2 cups mixed salad greens (such as lettuce, spinach, arugula)
* 1/2 cup cherry tomatoes, halved
* 1/4 cup sliced cucumbers
* 1/4 cup sliced bell peppers
* 1/4 cup shredded carrots
* 2 tablespoons balsamic vinaigrette dressing

Instructions:

* In a large bowl, toss together mixed salad greens, cherry tomatoes, cucumbers, bell peppers, and shredded carrots.
* Arrange sliced grilled chicken breast on top of the salad.
* Drizzle with balsamic vinaigrette dressing.
* Toss gently to combine all ingredients.

* Serve immediately as a light and satisfying lunch
option.

Health Benefits:

* This grilled chicken salad is rich in lean protein,
vitamins, and fiber, promoting satiety and supporting
overall health.

Preparation Time: 15 minutes

2. Lentil Soup

Ingredients:

* 1 cup dried lentils, rinsed
* 4 cups vegetable broth
* 1 onion, chopped
* 2 carrots, diced
* 2 celery stalks, diced
* 2 garlic cloves, minced
* 1 teaspoon dried thyme
* Salt and pepper to taste
* Fresh parsley for garnish

Instructions:

* In a large pot, heat olive oil over medium heat.

* Add chopped onion, carrots, and celery. Sauté until vegetables are softened.

* Stir in minced garlic and dried thyme, cook for another minute.

* Add rinsed lentils and vegetable broth to the pot.

* Bring to a boil, then reduce heat to simmer.

* Cover and cook for 25-30 minutes, or until lentils are tender.

* Season with salt and pepper to taste.

* Serve hot, garnished with fresh parsley.

Health Benefits:

* Lentils are rich in protein and fiber, while vegetables provide vitamins and minerals.

* This soup is hearty, nutritious, and filling.

Preparation Time: 40 minutes

3. Tuna Salad Wrap

Ingredients:

* 1 (5 oz) can tuna, drained

* 2 tablespoons Greek yogurt

* 1 tablespoon lemon juice

* 1/4 cup diced celery

* 1/4 cup diced red onion

* Salt and pepper to taste

* 2 whole wheat tortillas

* 1/2 cup mixed salad greens

Instructions:

* In a bowl, combine drained tuna, Greek yogurt, lemon juice, diced celery, and diced red onion.

* Season with salt and pepper to taste.

* Lay out whole wheat tortillas and place mixed salad greens on each.

* Spoon tuna salad mixture onto the center of each tortilla.

* Roll up tightly to form wraps.

* Slice in half diagonally and serve immediately.

Health Benefits:

* This tuna salad wrap is high in protein and omega-3 fatty acids, supporting heart health and providing essential nutrients.

Preparation Time: 10 minutes

4. Quinoa Salad with Chickpeas

Ingredients:

* 1 cup cooked quinoa
* 1 (15 oz) can chickpeas, drained and rinsed
* 1/2 cup diced cucumbers
* 1/2 cup halved cherry tomatoes
* 1/4 cup chopped red onion
* 1/4 cup chopped fresh parsley
* 2 tablespoons olive oil
* 1 tablespoon lemon juice
* Salt and pepper to taste

Instructions:

* In a large bowl, combine cooked quinoa, chickpeas, diced cucumbers, halved cherry tomatoes, chopped red onion, and chopped fresh parsley.
* In a small bowl, whisk together olive oil, lemon juice, salt, and pepper to make the dressing.
* Pour dressing over the quinoa salad mixture and toss to coat evenly.
* Serve chilled or at room temperature as a nutritious and flavorful lunch option.

Health Benefits:

* This quinoa salad is rich in plant-based protein, fiber, and vitamins, promoting satiety and supporting digestion.

Preparation Time: 20 minutes

5. Turkey and Avocado Wrap

Ingredients:

* 4 slices deli turkey
* 1/2 avocado, sliced
* 1/4 cup shredded lettuce

* 2 tablespoons hummus

* 2 whole wheat tortillas

Instructions:

* Lay out whole wheat tortillas and spread hummus evenly on each.

* Place shredded lettuce on top of the hummus layer.

* Arrange deli turkey slices and avocado slices on each tortilla.

* Roll up tightly to form wraps.

* Slice in half diagonally and serve immediately.

Health Benefits:

* This turkey and avocado wrap offers lean protein, healthy fats, and fiber, supporting muscle health and providing essential nutrients.

Preparation Time: 10 minutes

6. Veggie Stir-Fry with Tofu

Ingredients:

* 1/2 block extra-firm tofu, drained and cubed

* 1 tablespoon soy sauce

* 1 tablespoon sesame oil

* 1 teaspoon minced ginger

* 2 garlic cloves, minced

* 1 cup mixed vegetables (such as bell peppers, broccoli, carrots, snap peas)

* Cooked brown rice for serving

Instructions:

* In a bowl, marinate tofu cubes in soy sauce for 10 minutes.

* Heat sesame oil in a skillet over medium heat.

* Add minced ginger and garlic, sauté until fragrant.

* Add marinated tofu cubes to the skillet and cook until golden brown on all sides.

* Stir in mixed vegetables and cook until tender-crisp.

* Serve hot over cooked brown rice as a flavorful and satisfying lunch option.

Health Benefits:

* This veggie stir-fry with tofu is rich in plant-based protein, vitamins, and minerals, supporting overall health and providing energy.

Preparation Time: 20 minutes

7. Caprese Salad

Ingredients:

* 1 large tomato, sliced
* 1/2 cup fresh mozzarella cheese, sliced
* Fresh basil leaves
* 1 tablespoon balsamic glaze
* Salt and pepper to taste

Instructions:

* Arrange tomato slices and fresh mozzarella cheese slices on a serving plate.
* Tuck fresh basil leaves between the tomato and cheese slices.
* Drizzle with balsamic glaze.
* Season with salt and pepper to taste.
* Serve immediately as a light and refreshing lunch option.

Health Benefits:

*   This Caprese salad provides calcium, vitamin C, and antioxidants, supporting bone health and boosting immunity.

Preparation Time: 10 minutes

8. Chicken and Vegetable Stir-Fry

Ingredients:

*   1 boneless, skinless chicken breast, thinly sliced
*   1 tablespoon soy sauce
*   1 tablespoon oyster sauce
*   1 tablespoon olive oil
*   1 teaspoon minced garlic
*   1 cup mixed vegetables (such as bell peppers, snap peas, carrots, broccoli)
*   Cooked brown rice for serving

Instructions:

*   In a bowl, marinate chicken breast slices in soy sauce and oyster sauce for 10 minutes.
*   Heat olive oil in a skillet over medium-high heat.

* Add minced garlic and sauté until fragrant.

* Add marinated chicken breast slices to the skillet and cook until browned and cooked through.

* Stir in mixed vegetables and cook until tender-crisp.

* Serve hot over cooked brown rice as a flavorful and nutritious lunch option.

Health Benefits:

* This chicken and vegetable stir-fry provides lean protein, fiber, and essential nutrients, supporting muscle health and digestion.

Preparation Time: 20 minutes

9. Spinach and Feta Stuffed Bell Peppers

Ingredients:

* 2 bell peppers, halved and seeds removed

* 2 cups fresh spinach leaves

* 1/4 cup crumbled feta cheese

* 2 tablespoons olive oil

* 1 teaspoon minced garlic

* Salt and pepper to taste

Instructions:

* Preheat the oven to 375°F (190°C).
* In a skillet, heat olive oil over medium heat.
* Add minced garlic and sauté until fragrant.
* Add fresh spinach leaves and cook until wilted.
* Stir in crumbled feta cheese and season with salt and pepper to taste.
* Stuff each bell pepper half with the spinach and feta mixture.
* Place stuffed bell peppers on a baking sheet lined with parchment paper.
* Bake in the preheated oven for 20-25 minutes, or until bell peppers are tender.
* Serve hot as a delicious and nutritious lunch option.

Health Benefits:

* These spinach and feta stuffed bell peppers are rich in vitamins, minerals, and antioxidants, supporting overall health and immunity.

Preparation Time: 30 minutes

10. Egg Salad Lettuce Wraps

Ingredients:

* 4 hard-boiled eggs, chopped

* 2 tablespoons Greek yogurt

* 1 tablespoon Dijon mustard

* 1 tablespoon chopped chives or green onions

* Salt and pepper to taste

* Lettuce leaves for wrapping

Instructions:

* In a bowl, combine chopped hard-boiled eggs, Greek yogurt, Dijon mustard, and chopped chives.

* Season with salt and pepper to taste.

* Spoon egg salad mixture onto lettuce leaves.

* Roll up lettuce leaves to form wraps.

* Serve immediately as a light and protein-rich lunch option.

Health Benefits:

* These egg salad lettuce wraps are rich in protein and essential nutrients, supporting muscle health and providing energy.

Preparation Time: 15 minutes

Gout Diet Dinner Recipes for Seniors

1. Grilled Lemon Herb Chicken

Ingredients:

* 2 boneless, skinless chicken breasts
* 2 tablespoons olive oil
* 1 tablespoon lemon juice
* 1 teaspoon dried thyme
* 1 teaspoon dried rosemary
* Salt and pepper to taste

Instructions:

* Preheat grill to medium-high heat.
* In a small bowl, whisk together olive oil, lemon juice, thyme, rosemary, salt, and pepper.
* Brush the chicken breasts with the marinade on both sides.
* Grill chicken for 6-8 minutes per side, or until cooked through and juices run clear.
* Remove from grill and let rest for a few minutes before serving.

* Serve with steamed vegetables or a side salad for a complete meal.

Health Benefits:

* Grilled chicken is a lean protein source, while herbs and lemon juice add flavor without extra calories or purines.

Preparation Time: 20 minutes

2. Baked Salmon with Asparagus

Ingredients:

* 2 salmon fillets
* 1 bunch asparagus, trimmed
* 2 tablespoons olive oil
* 2 cloves garlic, minced
* 1 teaspoon lemon zest
* Salt and pepper to taste
* Fresh dill for garnish (optional)

Instructions:

* Preheat oven to 400°F (200°C).

* Place salmon fillets and asparagus on a baking sheet lined with parchment paper.

* In a small bowl, mix together olive oil, minced garlic, lemon zest, salt, and pepper.

* Brush the mixture over the salmon and asparagus.

* Bake for 12-15 minutes, or until salmon is cooked through and flakes easily with a fork.

* Garnish with fresh dill if desired before serving.

Health Benefits:

* Salmon is rich in omega-3 fatty acids, promoting heart health, while asparagus provides fiber and vitamins.

Preparation Time: 20 minutes

3. Turkey Meatballs with Zucchini Noodles

Ingredients:

* 1 lb ground turkey

* 1/4 cup breadcrumbs (use gluten-free if desired)

* 1 egg

* 2 cloves garlic, minced

* 1 teaspoon dried oregano

* 1/2 teaspoon dried basil

* Salt and pepper to taste

* 2 zucchinis, spiralized into noodles

* 1 cup marinara sauce

* Grated Parmesan cheese for serving (optional)

Instructions:

* Preheat oven to 400°F (200°C).

* In a bowl, combine ground turkey, breadcrumbs, egg, minced garlic, dried oregano, dried basil, salt, and pepper. Mix well.

* Shape the mixture into meatballs and place them on a baking sheet lined with parchment paper.

* Bake meatballs in the preheated oven for 15-20 minutes, or until cooked through.

* While the meatballs are baking, heat marinara sauce in a saucepan over medium heat.

* Add zucchini noodles to the saucepan and cook for 2-3 minutes until heated through but still crisp.

* Serve turkey meatballs with zucchini noodles, topped with grated Parmesan cheese if desired.

Health Benefits:

* Turkey is a lean protein source, while zucchini noodles offer a low-carb alternative to pasta, reducing purine intake.

Preparation Time: 30 minutes

4. Lentil Soup

Ingredients:

* 1 cup dried green lentils
* 1 onion, chopped
* 2 carrots, chopped
* 2 stalks celery, chopped
* 2 cloves garlic, minced
* 4 cups vegetable broth
* 1 teaspoon dried thyme
* 1 teaspoon dried rosemary
* Salt and pepper to taste
* Fresh parsley for garnish (optional)

Instructions:

* Rinse lentils under cold water and drain.

* In a large pot, heat olive oil over medium heat.

* Add chopped onion, carrots, celery, and minced garlic. Sauté for 5-7 minutes until vegetables are softened.

* Add lentils, vegetable broth, dried thyme, dried rosemary, salt, and pepper to the pot. Stir to combine.

* Bring the soup to a boil, then reduce heat to low and simmer for 25-30 minutes, or until lentils are tender.

* Taste and adjust seasoning if needed.

* Serve hot, garnished with fresh parsley if desired.

Health Benefits:

* Lentils are rich in fiber and protein, promoting satiety and digestive health.

* Vegetables add vitamins and minerals.

Preparation Time: 40 minutes

5. Quinoa Stuffed Bell Peppers

Ingredients:

* 4 bell peppers, tops removed and seeds removed

* 1 cup cooked quinoa

* 1 can (15 oz) black beans, drained and rinsed

* 1 cup corn kernels (fresh, frozen, or canned)

* 1 cup diced tomatoes

* 1/2 cup diced onion

* 2 cloves garlic, minced

* 1 teaspoon chili powder

* 1 teaspoon cumin

* Salt and pepper to taste

* Shredded cheese for topping (optional)

* Fresh cilantro for garnish (optional)

Instructions:

* Preheat oven to 375°F (190°C).

* In a large bowl, mix together cooked quinoa, black beans, corn kernels, diced tomatoes, diced onion, minced garlic, chili powder, cumin, salt, and pepper.

* Spoon the quinoa mixture into each bell pepper until they are filled to the top.

* Place stuffed bell peppers in a baking dish and cover with aluminum foil.

* Bake in the preheated oven for 25-30 minutes, or until bell peppers are tender.

* Remove foil and sprinkle shredded cheese on top of each bell pepper.

* Return to the oven and bake for an additional 5 minutes, or until cheese is melted and bubbly.

* Garnish with fresh cilantro before serving.

Health Benefits:

* This dish is packed with fiber and plant-based protein from quinoa and black beans, supporting digestive health and muscle maintenance.

Preparation Time: 45 minutes

6. Chicken Stir-Fry with Vegetables

Ingredients:

* 2 boneless, skinless chicken breasts, thinly sliced

* 2 cups mixed vegetables (such as bell peppers, broccoli, carrots, snap peas)

* 2 cloves garlic, minced

* 1 tablespoon ginger, minced

* 2 tablespoons soy sauce (use low-sodium if desired)

* 1 tablespoon olive oil

* Salt and pepper to taste

* Cooked brown rice for serving

Instructions:

* Heat olive oil in a large skillet or wok over medium-high heat.
* Add minced garlic and ginger, and sauté for 1 minute until fragrant.
* Add sliced chicken breasts to the skillet and cook until browned and cooked through, about 5-6 minutes.
* Add mixed vegetables to the skillet and stir-fry for 3-4 minutes until crisp-tender.
* Drizzle soy sauce over the chicken and vegetables, and toss to coat evenly.
* Season with salt and pepper to taste.
* Serve chicken stir-fry over cooked brown rice.

Health Benefits:

* This stir-fry is loaded with lean protein from chicken and fiber-rich vegetables, providing a balanced and nutritious meal for seniors.

Preparation Time: 25 minutes

7. Spinach and Mushroom Quiche

Ingredients:

* 1 store-bought or homemade pie crust

* 4 eggs

* 1 cup milk (dairy or plant-based)

* 1 cup chopped spinach

* 1 cup sliced mushrooms

* 1/2 cup shredded cheese (such as Swiss or Gruyere)

* 1/4 cup diced onion

* 2 cloves garlic, minced

* Salt and pepper to taste

* Cooking spray

Instructions:

* Preheat oven to 375°F (190°C).

* Roll out pie crust and press into a pie dish. Trim off any excess dough.

* In a skillet, heat cooking spray over medium heat.

* Add diced onion and minced garlic, and sauté until softened.

* Add chopped spinach and sliced mushrooms to the skillet, and cook until spinach wilts and mushrooms are tender.

* In a bowl, whisk together eggs, milk, salt, and pepper.

* Spread cooked vegetables evenly in the pie crust, then sprinkle shredded cheese on top.

* Pour egg mixture over the vegetables and cheese in the pie crust.

* Bake in the preheated oven for 35-40 minutes, or until the quiche is set and golden brown on top.

* Remove from oven and let it cool slightly before slicing.

* Serve warm or at room temperature.

Health Benefits:

* This quiche is rich in protein from eggs and calcium from cheese, while spinach and mushrooms add vitamins and antioxidants.

Preparation Time: 1 hour

8. Shrimp and Vegetable Stir-Fry

Ingredients:

*   1 lb shrimp, peeled and deveined

*   2 cups mixed vegetables (such as bell peppers, snap
    peas, carrots, broccoli)

*   2 cloves garlic, minced

*   1 tablespoon ginger, minced

*   2 tablespoons soy sauce (use low-sodium if desired)

*   1 tablespoon olive oil

*   Salt and pepper to taste

*   Cooked brown rice for serving

Instructions:

*   Heat olive oil in a large skillet or wok over medium-
    high heat.

*   Add minced garlic and ginger, and sauté for 1-minute
    until fragrant.

*   Add shrimp to the skillet and cook until pink and
    opaque, about 2-3 minutes per side. Remove from
    skillet and set aside.

*   Add mixed vegetables to the skillet and stir-fry for 3-
    4 minutes until crisp-tender.

* Return cooked shrimp to the skillet and toss with vegetables.

* Drizzle soy sauce over the shrimp and vegetables, and toss to coat evenly.

* Season with salt and pepper to taste.

* Serve shrimp and vegetable stir-fry over cooked brown rice.

Health Benefits:

* This stir-fry is packed with protein from shrimp and fiber-rich vegetables, providing a balanced and nutritious meal for seniors.

Preparation Time: 20 minutes

9. Eggplant Parmesan

Ingredients:

* 1 large eggplant, sliced into rounds

* 1 cup whole wheat breadcrumbs (use gluten-free if desired)

* 2 eggs, beaten

* 1 cup marinara sauce

* 1 cup shredded mozzarella cheese

* 1/4 cup grated Parmesan cheese

* 2 tablespoons chopped fresh basil

* Salt and pepper to taste

* Cooking spray

Instructions:

* Preheat oven to 375°F (190°C).

* Dip eggplant slices in beaten eggs, then coat with breadcrumbs.

* Place breaded eggplant slices on a baking sheet lined with parchment paper.

* Spray eggplant slices with cooking spray and bake in the preheated oven for 15-20 minutes, or until golden brown and tender.

* Spread marinara sauce evenly in a baking dish.

* Arrange baked eggplant slices over the marinara sauce.

* Sprinkle shredded mozzarella cheese and grated Parmesan cheese over the eggplant slices.

* Return to the oven and bake for another 10-15 minutes, or until cheese is melted and bubbly.

* Remove from oven and garnish with chopped fresh basil before serving.

Health Benefits:

* This eggplant parmesan is a healthier twist on the classic Italian dish, providing fiber from eggplant and calcium from cheese.

Preparation Time: 45 minutes

10. Cauliflower Fried Rice

Ingredients:

* 1 head cauliflower, riced
* 2 eggs, beaten
* 1 cup mixed vegetables (such as peas, carrots, corn)
* 2 cloves garlic, minced
* 2 tablespoons soy sauce (use low-sodium if desired)
* 1 tablespoon sesame oil
* 2 green onions, thinly sliced
* Salt and pepper to taste
* Cooking spray

Instructions:

* In a skillet, heat cooking spray over medium heat.
* Add beaten eggs to the skillet and scramble until cooked through. Remove from skillet and set aside.
* Add minced garlic to the skillet and sauté for 1 minute until fragrant.
* Add mixed vegetables to the skillet and stir-fry for 3-4 minutes until crisp-tender.
* Stir in riced cauliflower and cook for another 3-4 minutes until cauliflower is heated through.
* Add cooked eggs back to the skillet and stir to combine.
* Drizzle soy sauce and sesame oil over the cauliflower mixture, and toss to coat evenly.
* Season with salt and pepper to taste.
* Garnish with sliced green onions before serving.

Health Benefits:

* This cauliflower fried rice is a low-carb alternative to traditional fried rice, providing fiber and vitamins from cauliflower and vegetables.

Preparation Time: 25 minutes

Gout Diet Snacks Recipes for Seniors

1. Apple Slices with Peanut Butter

Ingredients:

* 1 apple, sliced

* 2 tablespoons peanut butter (or almond butter)

Instructions:

* Slice the apple into wedges or rounds.

* Spread peanut butter on each apple slice.

* Serve immediately as a satisfying and nutritious snack.

Health Benefits:

* Apples are rich in fiber and vitamin C, promoting digestion and immune health.

* Peanut butter provides healthy fats and protein, keeping you satisfied and providing energy.

2. Celery Sticks with Hummus

Ingredients:

* 2 celery stalks, cut into sticks
* 1/4 cup hummus

Instructions:

* Cut celery stalks into sticks.
* Dip celery sticks into hummus.
* Enjoy this crunchy and protein-rich snack.

Health Benefits:

* Celery is low in calories and high in fiber, aiding digestion and promoting satiety.
* Hummus offers protein and healthy fats, supporting muscle health and providing sustained energy.

3. Greek Yogurt with Granola

Ingredients:

* 1/2 cup Greek yogurt (plain or flavored)
* 1/4 cup granola
* 1 tablespoon honey or maple syrup (optional)

Instructions:

* Spoon Greek yogurt into a bowl.
* Sprinkle granola on top.
* Drizzle with honey or maple syrup if desired.
* Enjoy this creamy and crunchy snack.

Health Benefits:

* Greek yogurt is a good source of protein and probiotics, supporting gut health and immunity.
* Granola provides fiber and complex carbohydrates, offering sustained energy and keeping you full.

4. Trail Mix

Ingredients:

* 1/4 cup mixed nuts (such as almonds, walnuts, cashews)
* 2 tablespoons dried fruits (such as raisins, cranberries, apricots)
* 1 tablespoon dark chocolate chips or chunks

Instructions:

* Mix all ingredients together in a bowl.

* Portion into small snack bags for easy grab-and-go options.

* Enjoy this energy-boosting snack between meals.

Health Benefits:

* Nuts are rich in healthy fats, protein, and antioxidants, promoting heart health and reducing inflammation.

* Dried fruits offer natural sweetness and provide vitamins and minerals essential for overall health.

* Dark chocolate contains antioxidants and may improve mood and cognitive function.

5. Cottage Cheese with Pineapple

Ingredients:

* 1/2 cup low-fat cottage cheese
* 1/4 cup diced pineapple (fresh or canned in juice)

Instructions:

* Spoon cottage cheese into a bowl.
* Top with diced pineapple.

* Enjoy this sweet and savory snack packed with protein and vitamin C.

Health Benefits:

* Cottage cheese is high in protein and calcium, supporting muscle health and bone strength.
* Pineapple is rich in vitamin C and bromelain, aiding digestion and reducing inflammation.

6. Rice Cake with Avocado

Ingredients:

* 1 rice cake
* 1/4 avocado, sliced
* Pinch of salt and pepper

Instructions:

* Top rice cake with sliced avocado.
* Sprinkle with salt and pepper.
* Enjoy this simple and satisfying snack.

Health Benefits:

* Avocado provides healthy fats and fiber, keeping you full and promoting heart health.

* Rice cakes are low in calories and offer a crunchy texture, making them a satisfying snack option.

7. Veggie Sticks with Yogurt Dip

Ingredients:

* 1/2 cup mixed veggie sticks (such as carrots, cucumber, bell peppers)
* 1/4 cup Greek yogurt
* 1 tablespoon chopped fresh herbs (such as dill, parsley)
* Pinch of salt and pepper

Instructions:

* Arrange veggie sticks on a plate.
* Mix Greek yogurt with chopped herbs, salt, and pepper to make the dip.
* Serve veggie sticks with yogurt dip for a refreshing and crunchy snack.

Health Benefits:

* Mixed veggies are low in calories and high in fiber, vitamins, and minerals, supporting overall health and digestion.

* Greek yogurt provides protein and probiotics, promoting gut health and immunity.

8. Hard-Boiled Egg with Whole Grain Crackers

Ingredients:

* 1 hard-boiled egg
* 4 whole grain crackers

Instructions:

* Peel and slice the hard-boiled egg.
* Serve with whole grain crackers.
* Enjoy this protein-packed snack for a quick energy boost.

Health Benefits:

* Eggs are a complete protein source and contain essential vitamins and minerals, supporting muscle health and brain function.
* Whole grain crackers offer fiber and complex carbohydrates, providing sustained energy and keeping you full.

9. Cherry Tomato Caprese Skewers

Ingredients:

* 6 cherry tomatoes
* 6 mini mozzarella balls
* Fresh basil leaves
* Balsamic glaze (optional)

Instructions:

* Thread cherry tomatoes, mini mozzarella balls, and fresh basil leaves onto skewers.
* Drizzle with balsamic glaze if desired.
* Enjoy these colorful and flavorful skewers as a light and refreshing snack.

Health Benefits:

* Cherry tomatoes are rich in antioxidants and vitamin C, supporting immune health and reducing inflammation.
* Mozzarella balls provide protein and calcium, promoting muscle and bone health.

10. Cucumber Slices with Tzatziki

Ingredients:

* 1/2 cucumber, sliced
* 1/4 cup tzatziki sauce

Instructions:

* Arrange cucumber slices on a plate.
* Serve with tzatziki sauce for dipping.
* Enjoy this cool and creamy snack packed with vitamins and probiotics.

Health Benefits:

* Cucumbers are low in calories and high in water content, promoting hydration and aiding digestion.
* Tzatziki sauce contains probiotics and healthy fats, supporting gut health and providing satiety.

CONCLUSION

This Gout Diet Cookbook for Seniors serves as a comprehensive guide to managing gout effectively through delicious and nutritious recipes tailored to the unique dietary needs of seniors. By adhering to the principles of the gout diet, including limiting high-purine foods, focusing on low-purine options, staying hydrated, and maintaining a healthy weight, seniors can alleviate pain, reduce inflammation, and improve overall well-being.

With a wide array of breakfast, snack, lunch, dinner, and dessert options, this cookbook offers seniors flavorful meals that prioritize health without compromising on taste. Each recipe is carefully crafted to incorporate anti-inflammatory ingredients, promote hydration, and provide essential nutrients vital for managing gout and supporting overall health.

By following the guidelines and incorporating these recipes into their daily routine, seniors can take proactive steps towards managing their gout condition, reducing the frequency and severity of flare-ups, and enjoying a higher quality of life.